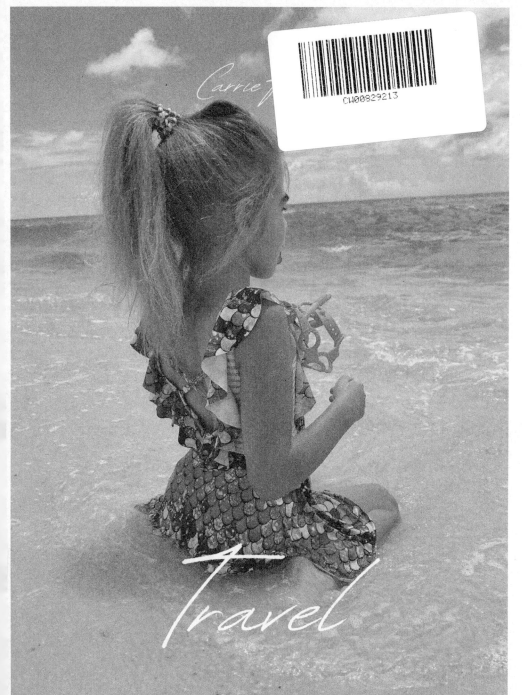

Carrie

Travel

Haidyn's Way

TRAVEL HAIDYN'S WAY

Our family's journey of traveling with a child with a disability and terminal illness.

Author & Mother:
Carrie Fowler

To my daughter, Haidyn.

Thank you for teaching me what the true meaning of unconditional love is. I may not be able to change your diagnosis or the hardships you face, but I vow to change the world in honor of you.
I love you.
Forever & for always,
Mama

INTRODUCTION

"Are we taking the bounce house?" asked my husband as we planned a weekend trip away to the Blue Ridge Mountains in North Georgia.

"Are we going to be able to fit all of this and did you let the host know that we may have to rearrange the Airbnb for safety?" he continued with a little concern and fair share of anxiety.

"Yes, we have to. We must create a safe space in the cabin for Haidyn. Otherwise, she will be miserable while we are enjoying our stay and not out adventuring during the day. I will message the host and let them know but if it's a problem then we will cancel, I guess." I said.

The conversation continued with more questions and concerns about traveling as a family of four, with an extra friend of our oldest daughter, three dogs and what seemed like an immeasurable number of items to pack. Nothing about this was normal and it was in that conversation filled with anxiety about all the worst things that could happen while away from the comfort of our home, we realized that if we wanted to create these memories for our children, in the short amount of time we had with our Haidyn then we would have to wing it in the outside world that isn't always accessible and inclusive of her needs.

Why were we intimidated? We had been winging it for months now.

Since Haidyn's diagnosis of Sanfilippo Syndrome in March of 2020, (YES, in the middle of the initial, Covid shutdown) we caught on quickly that we would be winging it through the medical world of having a child with a rare and terminal disease.

Her pediatrician had never heard of her diagnosis and many medical professionals we encountered knew little to nothing more. We were in a race against the clock of a short, life expectancy. We had much to learn, emotions to navigate and memories to create before it was too late.

The little glimmer of community with some knowledge was a small, Facebook group of parents of children with Sanfilippo Syndrome.

"What Is Sanfilippo Syndrome?

Imagine Alzheimer's & dementia, but in children.

In a nutshell, that's what every family of children with Sanfilippo Syndrome faces. Sanfilippo Syndrome, also known as Mucopolysaccharidosis type III is a terminal, neurodegenerative, rare disease. It causes children to lose all the skills they have gained, suffer seizures and movement disorders, experience pain and suffering, and then die, often before the second decade of life. Because of its neurodegenerative nature and multi-system impact, Sanfilippo Syndrome is often called, "Childhood Alzheimer's." Currently there is no FDA-approved treatment or cure. But there is hope."

-Cure Sanfilippo Foundation
CureSFF.org

I am writing this book in hopes that with sharing a small part of our family's journey of traveling with a medically complex child, I may be able to provide some tips, advice and inspiration to other families like ours that want to travel and create memories for their children despite the struggles and limitations of living in a world that is much unlike you and unprepared for you.

My family and I understand that each family's experiences and situations are unique. We are blessed in more ways than we can imagine despite the difficulties life has placed on our shoulders. We know that there are many families in a similar situation as us that may not have all that we do. We share our journey with humility, love, and empathy for each one of you.

We hope that whether you have more or less, or simpler or more complex journeys, that you feel that we are like you. We see you. We are proud of you, and we advocate for change for you, too.

Each of us are facing a world that has come so far and yet, still has an incredible amount of work, understanding and change needed in the lives of those with disabilities, high needs, rare diseases, and terminal illnesses.

Let us remember, we are a team. Knowledge is power and no one holds more power than us as parents and caregivers to advocate, educate and create change in this world for each other, our children, and our loved ones.

TO LEARN MORE ABOUT
Sanfilippo
Syndrome

You can follow our journey on
TikTok, Instagram & Facebook

@HAIDYNSHOPE

For more about ongoing research, education, meet the families or to donate.

CURE SANFILIPPO
FOUNDATION

@CURESANFILIPPO

CURESFF.ORG

UNIQUE NEEDS

As Haidyn's mama and full-time caregiver, I understand that her needs are exactly that. HER needs. She may have many things in common with other children that have the diagnosis of Sanfilippo Syndrome, but she will also have her own preferences, wants, quirks and personality traits.
As we prepare to travel, I must take into consideration how each vacation could possibly affect her

both positively and negatively. I am always overpacking and preparing for the worst-case scenario while hoping for the best. Amid that I have also taken on the mindset of, "it is what it is." One of the more difficult mindset shifts I have had to make on this journey with Haidyn is that no matter what, sometimes, it is what it is, and I have no control over the situation and lack the ability to be able to fix it.

I have no control over whether she will have a good day or a difficult day. With "neurological storms" as I like to call them, every single day is unpredictable, and the good days and bad days play an equal role in each week of her life.

I do have control over other things such as packing medications that help provide relief on the hard days and those needed for her daily intake. I can prepare for her sensory needs with her favorite toys, distractions, and weighted blankets. I prepare and pack all medical supplies and equipment for G-tube feeds, emergency kits, diapers, wipes and clothing for each day.

If you are like me and your child is like my Haidyn, you consistently pack a minimum of three outfits for every single outing or day that you will be away from home. Why? Because this beautiful girl never ceases to surprise me with the messes she can make or sudden, external out-puts from the inside of her cute, little body.

I have the ability to prepare for her mobility needs with packing a medical stroller, activity chair, AFOs (feet braces), a travel sleep safe bed, soft landings for a safe space, and more. I know, you are wondering how we pack all these things, and we will cover that too.

Most importantly, I want you to remember that your child's needs are their own. Pay no attention to anyone who tells you otherwise and accept with an open heart that how traveling looks for your family may not look the same as everyone else you know.

It may look like a whole lot on the outside. It may look like you've overpacked and over-prepared. It may look like exhaustion and stress. It may look like you are moving a small family cross country for a weekend. Yes, it feels like that too.

All that matters most is that you want to travel and make memories with your family in YOUR OWN WAY and you have the right to do so.

So, follow me and face the stress of overpacking to be able to enjoy the moments of traveling.

As you are forming a mental list or jotting one down on the back of the water bill, ask yourself these questions.

-What are my child's most complex needs and how will they impact our travel?

-What can I do to offset the impact of travel with these needs?

- Which medical needs must I provide for while we travel?

-Have I refilled medications, or will I be able to pick up from a local pharmacy while away if needed?

-What equipment is essential to take for safety to meet the mobility needs of my child?

-What sensory requirements must be met for my child daily and what can I pack for this?

-Where will my child sleep safely? Or do I need to provide a safer option so that I too can hopefully get some shut eye?

-Do I need to take into consideration of the closest emergency room/hospital?

-Would it be best to rent a condominium, Airbnb, home, or hotel room? (Camping, etc.)

-Should I pack safety items such as baby gates, door/oven locks, or harness/vest for my child?

-Will there be access to an elevator if needed for stroller/wheelchair?

-What do I need to pack regarding bathing/hygiene? (Bath chair, etc.)

-Should the weather keep us from leaving the residence, what can I pack to pass the time for my child in a new place? (iPad, DVD player, favorite toys, etc.)

-What additional supplies do I need, and do I need extra? (Formula, feed bags, emergency kits, etc.)

-What do I need to take for my self-care and time to decompress? (If allowed by your child, LOL!)

I hope this list of questions helps provide you with a better breakdown of what you need to prepare for your trip. As stated above, your family and your child's needs are specific to YOU.

Haidyn's needs are always evolving and ever changing. Sanfilippo Syndrome has slowly taken one ability to the next from her over the course of several years. She went from a child that could talk, sing her favorite songs, walk, run and play, to a child that can no longer do any of these things. She now has many health issues that affect her daily.

These consist of seizures, autonomic dysfunction, neurological storms, and even going days without sleep. From one vacation to the next, we are always reassessing what has changed and what we need to change for her. We had to accept to the best of our ability that we must make the accommodations to travel while we can before it is no longer possible for her or with her.

Thankfully, Haidyn is still able to travel and loves to visit new places even if it's extra work on our part and takes her a little more time to process.

We are grateful for every moment we have with her, and we want to continue to give her the absolute most out of life. Though not every vacation has been easy; it has been worth it to see her smile and be a part of memories that will last forever. She has taught us through her unique needs and complex medical journey, that we can still lead a beautiful life. We can continue to live in the moment with humility, empathy for others and a strength we did not know we had until we were gifted with her.

PLANNING & PREPARATION

"We need a cabin on a slab so that we can roll her in via her wheelchair, right?" I asked my husband.

"Or a cabin with minimal steps as possible so that we can carry her inside easily." He replied to me.

We are fortunate to be able to lift Haidyn and all her equipment when we must. We both try to do so as often as we can to stay strong and continue to be able to for as long as humanly possible, but as we get older and as she grows bigger this consistently becomes more of a challenge for us and we must take into consideration everyone's safety.

This comes in to play when we are being mindful of packing and unloading as well.

When it comes to our family and where we stay while on vacation, I prefer to stay in an Airbnb or vacation home. This is for several reasons. We enjoy the privacy and feel of a home versus a hotel room or condo. We pack A LOT to go anywhere with Haidyn and find it easier to pack, unload and set up inside of a home with a little more space and less people to worry about working around. When I stated that we pack A LOT, I meant it. We bring a majority of her equipment, a bounce house and lots of soft toys and landings to create a safe space for her within the home. We typically take two vehicles and a small trailer (depending on the trip and how long of a stay) to be able to bring everything needed, plus us and our dogs. One dog being Haidyn's service dog.

Before we do anything else to prepare for the trip, I start by spending a few days to a few weeks searching through multiple vacation home websites and viewing all the pictures of each home. This helps me gain more knowledge of the space, layout and possibility of creating a safe space for Haidyn while we are visiting. I am also searching for at least one king size bed in case she ends up in the bed with us one night or the entire time. Yes, we do pack a sleep safe bed made for traveling but sometimes, she makes her own rules about how sleep is going to play out for all of us.

A few focal points I pay attention to while sifting through pictures and descriptions of homes are on the next page.

-How many beds do we need & is at least one a king size?

-Is the living area or another space in the home big enough to create a designated safe space (including a bounce house) for Haidyn?

-Will I be able to move dangerous items out of her reach and block off spaces I do not want her to access
even by scooting her little booty across the floor?

-Is there a washer and dryer? YES, IT IS A MUST! We will need one because we rarely go a night without her soaking through a diaper. She is on a diuretic medication for pressure issues.

-Is the entry/drive big enough to fit two large vehicles and a trailer?

-Is the home on a slab, have a ramp, minimal steps or easy to access?

-What are the bathrooms like?
Can I fit her bath chair in a tub
provided or does it have a walk-in
shower we can use?

-Is it pet friendly/child friendly?
Yes, there are some vacation
homes that do not allow children
and/or pets.

-Do we have space and privacy
from neighbors?

-What is the pet/cleaning fee?

-Should we need to leave early or cancel ahead of time, is there a refund/partial refund policy?

-How close is the home to places we want to visit while out like restaurants, scenery, parks, beaches, etc.? (Some days are hard for Haidyn when it comes to spending long durations in the car.)

-How close is the nearest hospital, children's hospital, or urgent care in case of emergency?

-Is there at least one TV with cable or Netflix for Haidyn to watch? (She can no longer operate her iPad but still enjoys watching cartoons.)

-Is there a local grocery store nearby for snacks, hygiene products and extras that we need for the stay? (Once we have arrived and unpacked one of us will typically make a store run.)

If I can find answers to the previous list of questions, then we are looking good to book. But before I book, I reach out to the host of the Airbnb/vacation home. I explain in lengthy detail about our family, our unique situation with Haidyn, our pets and any additional information or questions the host needs to know or can help answer for me.

By doing so, this will help prevent any last-minute issues or complaints coming from our stay. I inform the host of the limits and safety that are required to protect our daughter and provide her with a comfortable stay in their home. I let them know that I may move unsafe items from her reach temporarily and I may move furniture to create a safe space for her. I always assure the host that I will take pictures of the initial setup when we arrive and place everything back just the way I

found it before our departure. But if anything is not "just right" or I forgot where an item originally came from, I vow to leave it out in clear view for
someone to find and place back in its original state.

I assure the host that I want to protect their home and my daughter with equal value, and I will own up to and do what I can, should something in their home become broken or damaged during our stay. This has yet to happen, and I am crossing my fingers that it never does, but with a child like, Haidyn it's always a possibility. I let them know how grateful I am to have the opportunity and option to do this with her. I share that I am happy to answer their questions as they answer mine. I also welcome the idea of a review on my Airbnb profile for future hosts to see that I follow through with my promise to protect their home. This process may require different questions to be answered or a unique to you experience and that is perfectly fine. I share this to provide insight and advice if you are unsure of what to ask, where to begin or what your own limits may be with you and your child. It may be easier for you to stay in a hotel room or condominium than it is for my family. Haidyn going days without sleep and at times having a rough day, she can become extremely loud. LOUD. We choose privacy to keep our peace and to preserve the ears of others when we can help it. Remember, what works for you is best.

My favorite travel platform to book with is Airbnb but there are many others you can find access to via a quick google search. My main advice is to make sure there are up to date pictures of the layout of the home and a beneficial description of rules, expectations of the host and other offers the home provides. If you have additional questions and to protect your family for your stay, I always advise to reach out to the host or booking company and make sure nothing goes overlooked or unanswered via documentation like email, messenger, or text message. Save and screenshot that confirmation for an extra layer of protection because we have all heard a few horror stories.

My last piece of advice is to listen to your intuition about the booking. If you are a mama or caregiver to a child with a disability or medical complexities, then your gut probably led you to a diagnosis and much more to follow. Allow it to continue to guide you as you make choices that regard the safety and care of your child. Yes, even while traveling and booking a stay.

You have enough stress and anxiety to navigate daily in this life. If something feels wrong, it probably is, and we don't need to add more to our already overflowing plates if we can help it.

PS- remember to pack any medical documentation you may need for special assistance.

HOW ARE WE GETTING THERE?

Listen, I am going to be straight forward with you right now and say that I have zero advice on flying with Haidyn. To be honest, I am terrified to do so for multiple reasons and I will refuse to do so unless we have no choice. While many families have had good experiences flying with their disabled children, many of us have heard of the hardships of traveling with just an upset baby on a plane. Haidyn is loud and has no awareness of how her volume level may bother others. She also lacks impulse control and at times there is nothing we can do to console her. We must ride it out. While she deserves to hold space in this world, I also try to hold space for others around us when possible.

Could she do great on a plane? Absolutely. Do I think she would? Probably not and I really do not want to find out the hard way. We can call this another episode of protecting my peace as the mother and caregiver of a disabled child. Therefore, when it comes to transportation we prefer to drive. For us that looks like loading up my suburban and my husband's truck with a trailer attached.

This does cost us more in fuel and miles on our vehicles, but it works for us. We can stop and get out for breaks when necessary and we can assure all our luggage will arrive safely. We have access to all of Haidyn's things whenever we need them, and she can yell at us the entire car ride if she would like. When it comes to what works best for your family, do that thing you do mama! If that is flying with more bravery than me, I applaud you. You are a badass!

If it looks like fitting in one or ten vehicles, do it. You may be able to rent a larger vehicle from a local dealership. We rent a small U-Haul when a trailer is necessary. Hop on google and search for vehicles or trailers for rent nearest you. Transportation comes in many forms and prices depending on the budget you have allowed and the vehicle of your choice. The most important aspect is what will provide the easiest travel for your child and the most peace in your pocket.

Do not worry about keeping up with the Jone's travel plans.

If you are considering flying, I have heard that a few airports offer special services for those with disabilities and special needs. We have not witnessed or tried this out as a family but have been told by friends that airports like Hartsfield-Jackson in Atlanta may allow you and your child to take a tour of the airport and even a plane before your trip to help with the transition for your child. If you are interested, I would consider looking into this being an option if it suits your family or eases some of you and your child's anxiety surrounding flying while traveling.

Follow your heart to make memories with your family.

ALL THE ACTIVITIES & SAFETY

We know our destination and we have booked the trip. I am not an overly organized or event planner of a mama. One of my best qualities is the ability of winging it, easily.

To me, vacation is about ditching the schedule, the routine, and the need to have a plan. I enjoy deciding what is for dinner right before we leave to try a new restaurant while out of town. But, with Haidyn I do have to create somewhat of a plan for activities, outings, and safety even on a relaxing vacation. Plus, once we have children, I believe we are just imagining that we are relaxing while on vacation. Reality is very much chaos & coordinating it the best we can. Fortunately, for me, Haidyn does not require an intense and set schedule to sustain happiness and adjust to the world around her. I understand that with your child this may look much different, and you will have to adjust accordingly to what benefits your child.

When planning activities for the trip I still take it day by day because I am able to with my family. We typically decide what we would like to do that day by discussing it the night before or the morning of. I will follow up with searching accessible places that make outings easier with Haidyn. This could be a park, nature preserve, beach, museum, or shopping. Many of these places will have accessible options for children like her in known tourist areas.

Another thing we like to do is to drive around the town we are staying in and site see. While doing this we can pick out a place that we would like to visit and that looks accessible for Haidyn. Worst case scenario is that it is too difficult, too much for Haidyn or it just plain out doesn't work, and we find a plan B.

We have learned to always be open to plan B, C, D or even E because if something can change, fall apart, or simply not work with Haidyn, it will most likely happen at least once. There is no sense in staying all worked up about it but instead moving forward and trying something new to continue enjoying our trip and making memories. Letting go of control and allowing change keeps us happier. As unique as our situation is, we cannot always plan for everything. There will be mishaps and the unexpected events. Shoot, that's our daily life with

Haidyn and we have little to no control of when things will go haywire - whether at home or away. The important thing is to always have a backup plan. Be ready for an emergency exit at any moment and do our absolute best to keep her safe wherever we may be. The rest is left unwritten and the best way to find the light in the dark is to quit focusing on controlling the narrative.

Life is short, weird, and hard. It never really goes the way we planned but that does not mean we cannot have a damn good time regardless!

What if the trip is a total failure? Everything goes wrong and nothing we planned for works out. Well, we have the ability to try again, and should she not be here before we try again then at least we tried in the first place. Life and travel are about getting out of your comfort zone. You must be willing to exit your comfort zone and make change to have the opportunity to make memories with your family. It is okay to have worries and anxiety about it. I would expect nothing less as a mama that feels all these things with you.

SAFETY.
NECESSITIES.
CONTROL WHAT YOU CAN,
BREATHE AND LET GO OF
THE REST.

CREATING A SAFE SPACE FOR HAIDYN

If you have followed us on social media platforms for a while, then you know that I have often gone viral for the safe room and spaces I have created for Haidyn within our home and while away on vacation.

As Sanfilippo Syndrome has stolen abilities from Haidyn, like mobility, her risk of falling and injury skyrocketed. As this progressed, I began making changes full of soft landings, safe toys to play with and a sensory friendly environment that was beneficial to Haidyn. I purchased a giant bounce house that she used to be able to climb up into and slide out of. Now, we place her at the top and she still wiggles down when she wants. At one point we had two bounce houses. I added puzzle piece, foam flooring with machine washable rugs on top to prevent some of the hurt from a fall or head bump on a concrete floor. I stocked up on gym mats and used tumble tracks that my oldest had from cheer for extra cushion. We slowly replaced any toys that became a danger or choking risk with both small and large, soft toys and stuffed animals. Firm storage bins and baskets were replaced with soft ones and there are baby gates to protect sharp corners and the TV. I added blankets over the tops of any furniture with sharp corners that were needed in the room. Paper and cardboard books were replaced with soft, washable, and indestructible books. She loves flipping through the pages and chewing on them occasionally. We share a giant bonus room/bedroom with Haidyn. Before she had her own bed, we combined her full-sized bed and our king-sized bed to create one giant bed for all of us to sleep comfortably. We continue to leave the beds like this for the rare occasion of when she ends up in bed with us. Plus, it is kind of cool and really comfy! We included giant bean bags to place strategically where she falls often when trying to stand or climb. She can no longer walk unassisted but continues to try and climb or stand on her own. YAY! GO BABY GIRL! She is my little warrior that refuses to give up.

Yes, it is a lot. A lot of stuff, change, reorganizing constantly and to clean but it is worth it!

HAIDYN'S STUFF
(FOR HOME & TRAVEL)

-Bounce House
(Walmart or Amazon)
-Bean Bags (Amazon)
-Medical Stroller
(Convaid Rodeo Tilt)
-Activity Chair with tray (Rifton)
-Soft Basket Assortment (Amazon)
-Weighted Blankets (Amazon)

-Foam Flooring (Amazon)
-Washable Rugs (Amazon)
-Giant Unicorn Stuffed Animal (Amazon)
-Indestructible Books (Amazon)
-Giant Pillows (Amazon)
-Gymax Trampoline for Bed (Amazon or Walmart)
-Japanese Floor Mattress (Amazon)
-Silicone Chewies (Amazon)
-Squishmallows (Amazon)
-Soft Ball Pit (Amazon)
-Baby Gates (Amazon)
-Wardrobes for Storage (Amazon)

-Care Bear Assortment (Amazon)
-Luggage bags for travel
(Amazon & the occasional trash
bag for convenience)
-Giant Diaper Bag (Amazon)
-Car seat (The Roosevelt)
-Travel Sleep Safe Bed
(SafePlaceBedding.com)
-Ski Vest/Harness for assisted
walking (Amazon)
-Outdoor Stroller
(Wonderfold Wagon)
-Seat for Wagon (Special
Tomato)
-DVD Player (Amazon)

-Noise Cancelling Headphones (Amazon)
-Winter Gloves to prevent hand chewing (Amazon)

This list covers many of the most commonly asked questions about "Haidyn's stuff." You may find the answer to more via our social media platforms. When it comes to Haidyn and her stuff, we take whatever we feel is necessary to provide the most comfort and easiest transition for her. This is why we often take two vehicles and a trailer to be able to accommodate her.

At first, it felt almost ridiculous to take all of this and spend extra in gas money. Let us add the time and planning it takes to pack and unpack it all. Yet, as we shifted through what navigating travel for OUR family looked like, we began to realize that it didn't matter how ridiculous it looked to others. What mattered most was Haidyn, her needs and finding ways to live in the moment that fit our lifestyle.

It never really was about the stuff. It has always been about her and for her. For us.

MORAL OF THE STORY

If you want to take the trip and
travel with your family despite the
obstacles of having a child with a
disability or terminal illness, do
NOT let the world stop you.
Your child deserves to hold space
in this world. You deserve to hold
space in this world. The picture of
what it was supposed to look like
in your head, that never existed.

You are creating that picture of what it is supposed to be like, now. If you cannot change it, you have the ability to make the best of every second you are given with your precious child. Do not let the need for control cause you to miss that.

"Life is uncontrollable, but when we let go, we find joy." -Carrie

I know that this book will not cover every obstacle that your family faces while traveling but if right now you

are paralyzed with fear and lacking the thought process of where to begin, I hope this brings you inspiration and a little advice. You are not alone. I was once you with no idea of what to do or where to turn and I just began to do what I do best and WING IT! It is going to be scary, and you are going to be anxious.
It is okay to feel all those hard emotions while preparing for change

with a disabled child. I don't claim to have all of the answers and I am embracing change daily, but I promise to share the little that I do know with others like me in hopes that maybe one day, we won't feel so alone on this journey.

ABOUT THE AUTHOR
Carrie Fowler

Carrie is the mother of two daughters and a wife to her husband, Caleb. While life has placed her in the unimaginable circumstances of navigating her youngest's journey with Sanfilippo Syndrome, she finds joy and passion in sharing her knowledge. She is an advocate for the Sanfilippo Syndrome community, the disability community, women's rights, and a life coach who specializes in grief and overcoming feeling stagnant in the dark. Through sharing her story and her daughter's story she hopes to enlighten others on how to find light in the darkest of moments.

She may not be able to save her daughter, but she vowed to tell the world her name, "Haidyn."

Printed in Great Britain
by Amazon

24602425R00046